MELISSA PRELL

The Nightshift Curse

How to Successfully Lose Weight While Working Nightshift

This book was professionally typeset on Reedsy.
Find out more at reedsy.com

Contents

1 Introduction   1

2 Night Shift Sucks!   5

3 When it is important, you find a way   9

    Creating a schedule   9

    Fitting in workouts   12

    Nutrition   13

    Stress Reduction   15

    Sleep Hygiene   16

    Family time   18

4 If I Can, So Can You!   19

Also by Melissa Prell   20

1

Introduction

o you find yourself wanting to lose weight but struggle to get started or stick to a plan long enough to start seeing results? Are you one of thousands who do shift work and can't find a way to make it work?

Shift work is simply working hours that are not your typical 9-5. Typically, the main shift that is referred to as shift work is an overnight shift. However, there are other shifts that are considered shift work and can make creating a healthy routine more difficult.

Some examples of shift work could be:

- 2 pm–10 pm, a swing shift
- 10 pm–6 am, a night shift
- 12 am–8 am, another night shift
- 4 pm–4 am, a 12hr swing shift into nights
- 8 pm–8 am, a 12hr night shift

When you look at these hours, you can see that they all play a role in disrupting your natural circadian rhythm, also known as your sleep cycle. When you start to disrupt that rhythm, it can throw many different aspects of your life off and make it more difficult to reach some of the goals that you might have.

It is not IMPOSSIBLE to reach your goals! In fact, it is very possible.

Now why should you listen to what I have to say and the advice in this book?

Because I am living it. I am going through it. I know the struggles that come with working a night shift, wanting to lose weight, and maximizing my time with my kids.

I am a nurse, and I work 8 pm–8 am. I am a mom of four amazing girls. I am a wife to a loving husband. I understand the struggle to lose weight and keep it off. In fact, I have been on the weight loss roller coaster for pretty much my entire life. Growing up, I was one of the "bigger" kids. Throughout my time in the military, I still struggled with losing weight and being at a weight that was acceptable for the army. I had my two oldest daughters while in the army in 2005 and 2009. Although they had a physical fitness program, it wasn't what I needed to be able to lose the weight and keep it off. I got deployed to Iraq twice and lost the weight during each deployment, only to regain it once I got back. Getting out of the army in 2011 didn't help either because I was going through a divorce and became a single mom of two girls. Still, I kept wanting to lose the weight!

Because of being on the weight loss roller coaster for so long, I knew all the wrong ways to lose weight and would always resort to them anytime I got on a "weight loss kick":

- Extreme intermittent fasting (such as eating one meal a day)
- Extreme calorie restrictions (often combined with extreme inter-mittent fasting)
- Exercising for hours every day
- Eliminating foods or food groups (because carbs are bad right?)

But I was missing some key components that would have helped me achieve the long-lasting weight loss I had been seeking for so long! However, I didn't even realize it until recently.

Fast forward to October 2021. I'm now working as a nurse, working night shift, and now have four girls. I found myself back in a position of wanting to lose weight, but I wanted to do it differently this time. Every other time I tried to lose weight, I would exercise more and restrict my eating. What I never did was change my relationship with food and change how I used food. You see, I had a negative relationship with food since I used it as a coping mechanism. I was an emotional eater. I ate out of boredom. I ate because of stress. So, this time I wanted to flip the script by starting with my nutrition.

I knew it wouldn't be easy, seeing that I had kids who don't necessarily like the veggies I like, and working the night shift made it harder to stay consistent with meals. Still, I was determined to find a way to make it work.

I was successful! Through small changes in how I ate, how I saw food, and how I used food, I was able to start losing weight without adding in exercise. This was something I didn't really think was possible, but here it was happening! Within the first two months, I was down about 15 pounds. Now that may not seem like a lot, but for someone who has always struggled, this was a huge success. Plus, it wasn't as hard as I thought it would be. Then I added in the exercise component. I made some further refinements to my nutrition and continued to lose weight. In total, so far, I have lost about 40-50 pounds.

It hasn't been perfect. It has been FAR from it! But I want to show you that through some simple changes, you can start seeing the results that you are looking for without starving yourself, without doing crazy amounts of exercise, and without having to eliminate some of your favorite foods! I also want you to know that even though working the night shift is hard, it is possible to be able to lose weight and keep it off.

All this information I am sharing is from the learning I have done, the experiences I have gone through on my journey, and what has worked for me. You will need to find what works for you, but this would be a good starting point.

2

Night Shift Sucks!

If you work the night shift, you probably agree! Night shift is hard. It makes it hard to do pretty much anything you want to do.

- Hard to spend time with family
- More difficult to schedule important appointments
- You constantly have an inconsistent sleep schedule/cycle
- Your nutrition becomes a struggle because you are tired all the time (or a lot of the time)
- Stress seems to become a normal part of your life because the issues with sleep and struggles with nutrition amplify any and all stress

It may even seem like there is no way to make it work, and all you want to do is scream! (Insert scream if needed, no judgment here)

Let's get into these different areas, and I'll explain why these are more difficult while working shift work.

Sleep

One of the biggest areas of your life that is affected by shift work is your sleep. This one is pretty easy to identify as an issue, but it is one of the more complicated problems to try to resolve without changing what shift you work. You work while everyone else is sleeping but then have days where you must try to function like a normal human being during the day, when you aren't working. You are going to bed at different times, depending on what your schedule is. Sometimes, your employer loves you so much that they only give you a single day off in between shifts. Then what? I have had this happen, and I absolutely HATE IT when they do this.

What happens when you have chronic sleep deprivation?

- Impaired cognition and memory
- Increased symptoms of depression as it disrupts the neurotransmitters that help regulate mood
- Increased risk of breast cancer
- Higher levels of anxiety
- Four times more likely to have a stroke when you sleep six hours or less a night
- Higher risk for heart disease
- Weight gain related to an imbalance in the hormones that make you feel hungry and full
- Higher risk for diabetes due to a lack of sleep increases cortisol, which can lead to insulin resistance

When you want to lose weight, you must find a way to maximize your sleep time and the quality of your sleep, so that you are able to reach your goals. I know that when I started my journey back in October 2021, sleep was something I prized and did not want to sacrifice. However, when I wanted to add in the exercise aspect, I knew that it was something that would help me to reach my goals. But how can I get as much sleep as I can while still being able to fit in exercise, family time, showering, eating, and getting out the door on time?

Family

We want to be able to spend time with family but work wacky hours. Kids have school activities they want you to be present for or extra-curricular activities they need you to drive them to and from during the week. But all these amazing things happen while you are sleeping or while you are working.

Unfortunately, there is no easy answer or fix to this one. It is easy to want to do all these things with your kids and family, but it is also important to be realistic about what you are truly capable of doing.

Stress

Even going through nursing school, I never really understood how stress could affect the body. But there is more than just emotional/mental stress. Your body goes through stress when you don't get enough sleep, when you do intense workouts, work long hours, and even do something as simple as change. Whenever our body is stressed, it releases a hormone called cortisol. While some cortisol is good and can be a source of energy, too much cortisol can cause you to gain weight, especially around the midsection. Too much cortisol can also cause damage to your adrenals and your hormone balance. If your hormone levels get all out of whack, it will be even harder to lose the weight and keep it off! Chronic stress can lead to even more serious health conditions, such as:

- Depression
- Heart disease
- Heart attacks (AKA myocardial infarctions)
- Fertility problems
- Skin disorders, such as eczema and psoriasis
- Diabetes

So how do we minimize stress and our body's response to stress so that we can lose the weight and keep it off?

Nutrition

This is one of the biggest struggles anyone has when trying to lose weight! You want to be able to lose weight, but you don't want to give up your pizza, pasta, and burgers. Or maybe you crave sweets and would rather keep your desserts, chocolate, and ice cream. Working the night shift makes it a little harder since your eating schedule gets out of whack, just like your sleep schedule. When do you eat breakfast? When is it best to eat a particular meal? What is the best plan for success when your schedule is so inconsistent?

I know that when I started my journey, I was concerned about when to eat a certain meal. This was something I had to figure out. It was harder for me to answer because I wanted to still be able to eat dinner with my family prior to going to work. So, it meant getting creative.

Schedule

You are given your work schedule. You take a look at it, and you wonder how you are going to be able to do the things you want to do to reach the goals that you want to reach. Sometimes, it seems like it is going to be impossible. I've been working night shift consistently for about three years, and there are still times when I must adapt the schedule I had created to my current circumstances. In other words, I make changes to how I do things based on circumstantial and temporary reasons. It isn't as hard as it may seem. Maybe a little overwhelming, but not difficult when you take it one step at a time.

3

When it is important, you find a way

If this is something that is truly important to you and it's a priority, you will find a way to make things happen. Like anything in life, what you focus on is what you will work on and what you will get results in. In this chapter, I will walk you through some of the different techniques and tactics that worked for me. Remember that you will need to adapt it to fit your schedule. What worked for me may not be what you need, but this is a great starting point.

Creating a schedule

When you want to start a weight loss plan or program, it is vital that you figure out your schedule and how you are going to fit stuff in from the very beginning. This schedule needs to be fixed enough that you don't change it regularly, but flexible enough to adjust when needed.

Step one

The first step is to simply put your work schedule onto a calendar. You can go old school and use paper (such as a planner or a calendar), or you can utilize digital calendars on your phone or computer. You can even create custom calendars and schedules on Microsoft Word. This is important because you need to start identifying where you have openings in your day. You also need to include any commute time and time to get ready for work, such as showering and packing the things you need for the shift.

Step two

The next step will be to insert your sleep time. This may seem odd to add to the schedule, but as you will find out, sleep is very important to your health, and you need to prioritize it! The goal is for you to get 7–8 hours of sleep every time you sleep. I realize that working the night shift means that you may not get a full 7–8 hours of rest, so get as much sleep as you can between shifts and make up for some of it when you are off.

Step three

Once you have those two things on the schedule, you will see some openings where you can start adding exercise time slots. Keep in mind that you do not need to exercise to lose weight and keep it off. As I have learned through my own journey, losing weight is mainly about the foods you eat, the quantities you eat, and when you are eating. Exercise can simply be seen as extra credit. To start off, maybe find three days each week that you can add in a workout.

Step four

Add anything else that needs to be added. This is when you can start to add in appointments, family activities, and other stuff.

Step five

You must figure out how you want to handle your days off. Do you want to continue to stay on a night shift schedule, regardless of if you are working or not? Do you want to switch yourself to days so that you can get stuff done? If you decide to switch to days during your days off, you then need to figure out how you are going to get your body back onto a night shift schedule.

How did I create my schedule?

This is what I did when I created my schedule, and this is what I still use. I work from 7:30 pm to 8:00 am, three to four days a week. I have a two-week block schedule, meaning I know what my schedule should be for each pay period. I have an hour's drive to and from work. It typically takes me about 30 minutes to shower, get dressed, and pack my stuff up. I also wanted to be able to have dinner with my family.

I worked backward from when I needed to leave, through the time that I needed to get ready, to the time I that had family dinner, to figure out what time I needed to be done working out (if I wanted to workout). That would then tell me what time I had to get up and do my workout to stay on schedule.

My sleep is always the same in between my shifts. I get home at about 9 am. I change out of my scrubs, and am in bed no later than 9:30 am. I get up between 3 pm and 3:30 pm, so that I can get my workout in. Because my workouts are important to me, I sacrifice a bit of sleep in order to get them done. On days I know that I will not workout, I will get up later to allow for a little more sleep. But I will still be up in time to have dinner with the family and get ready for work on time.

I personally wanted to be able to switch over to days so I could spend time with my kids on my days off. This is how I do it. This may work for you, and maybe it won't. You have to figure out what works for you. This is one area that I have changed because I realized I couldn't keep doing my original routine. When I get home, and I know I don't have to work that evening, I will nap for about two hours. What I used to do was stay up as long as I could, and then just go to sleep for the night with the goal of staying up until our family dinner. This stopped working for me, so I changed it to a two-hour nap. I will get up and stay awake until my kids go to bed between 8 pm and 9 pm. I will sometimes go to bed earlier, depending on how tired I am. The next day, I allow myself to sleep in and don't force myself to get up. No matter what, I am typically up by 7:30 am. Now when I need to switch back to nights, I will get up super early that morning, around 4:30 am. So, if I have to go back to work Monday evening, I will get up Monday morning at 4:30 am. I will stay up until 11 am, then lie down and take a nap until my normal wake up time of 3:00 pm to 3:30 pm.

Rinse and repeat.

Essentially, you have to find what works for your work schedule and your stage in life.

Fitting in workouts

For me, adding my workouts at the end of December 2021 was important to me. Even though I didn't "have" the time, I "made" the time to get it done. Was I tired? Yep. Am I glad I made it a priority, and did it anyway? Absolutely!

Fitting your workouts into your schedule will be based on what type of workout you want to do and if you have to go anywhere to do it, such as driving to a gym vs. doing a workout at home. If you have to drive to a gym, you will also need to consider that when making your schedule. This may deter you from doing as many workouts during the week since it takes longer to do them. Being able to do workouts from home simplifies it and allows you to go from your bed to your "gym" almost right away (after you change into your workout clothes and do your pre-workout, if you have a "gym" to use). I happen to have a small home gym that allows me to do bodyweight workouts, strength training with a variety of dumbbells, and cycling. If you don't have the equipment, that is ok too! There are so many different workouts that can be done without any other equipment other than your body.

Find the type of workout you want to do and then figure out when you want to fit it into the schedule.

Nutrition

This is the key! You can't skip this step and expect to have long-term success. You may have heard the phrase, "You can't out train a bad diet." If not, it simply means you can't workout to overcomes a poor diet. Your nutrition is the cornerstone of your health and longevity. It is truly the key to losing weight for good.

Now, I am not talking about having to be perfect or going on a crazy "diet," or eliminating foods or food groups. I do not like the word diet. To me, diet means it is temporary, and that is not what you are looking for. You are looking for long-term results, which means you have to be willing to make some lifelong changes to your nutrition.

There are a ton of different "diets" available on the internet. However, a lot of them are based on restriction and elimination. I've tried a lot of them, and they are hard to stick to. People have had great results with them. If you find one that works for you, that is what is important. I just prefer the nutrition plan that doesn't require me to give up double chocolate mug cakes or having pizza with my family when we have pizza night.

Here are some areas where you can make some easy, simple changes:

- **Eat more vegetables**. This one may seem obvious, but let me explain why it is important. Veggies are filled with fiber, which will help fill you up and keep you full. They are also packed with nutrients that your body needs to fully operate.
- **Drink more water**. Water is vital to health. Our bodies require water for pretty much everything, from energy production to the digestion of food. Water is also necessary to keep the body hydrated. More than likely, you are not drinking enough water. I always have a water bottle with me to help remind me to drink my water.

Quick tip: drink water when you think you are hungry. There are many times we mistake thirst for being hungry. Drink 10-12 oz of water and wait about 30 minutes. If it were thirst, the feeling would have started to go away. If it were truly hunger, it would help you to eat a little less as you have filled part of your stomach with water.

- **Try to eliminate processed foods**. This is going to be a bit harder since so much of our foods are processed. The goal is to eat more whole foods, or foods that are unaltered from plant to table. Processed foods have nutrients removed due to the nature of being processed, and a lot of them have other things added that are not necessarily good for our bodies. If you like bread, take a crack at making your own. It is actually way easier than you may think!
- **Plan your week in advance**. This was one thing that was a huge factor in my success. I planned our family dinners a week at a time. Some will plan all three meals for the week. That is not what I choose to do. What this also does is help you save money when you are grocery shopping. By knowing what you are having for dinner, it helps you to know what you will need to get from the store.

Quick tip: if you tend to pick up extra stuff when walking around the store, even if you have a list, do a pickup order from your favorite grocery store (if it is available). I do this ALL the time when I get groceries. I know I will have everything I need, and I don't spend money on things I don't actually need!

- **Eat slower!** Seriously, slow down. Eating is not a race. When you eat fast, you are not allowing your body to tell you when you are full so that you don't overeat. When you take a bite of food, put your fork/spoon down on the table and fully chew that bite before swallowing. Take time to have a conversation with your family.

When you slow down your eating, you may be surprised at how much less you eat.

- **Use small salad plates**. This may sound odd, but hear me out. Imagine you have two plates, one small and one big. You have two servings exactly the same size for the two plates. Each plate gets a serving. The small plate is filled, while the big plate has open areas. Even though the two plates have the same amount, our brains are going to think there isn't enough on the bigger plate. We "eat with our eyes" first, meaning what we see has a big impact on how we eat and how much we eat. When you look at the small plate that is full, the brain will believe that there is plenty of food. I use this trick myself and I can tell you that there is a difference. I find myself eating double when I use a large plate as compared to a small plate!

Stress Reduction

Reducing stress is important to your overall health and longevity. Chronic stress increases your risk for so many health problems. There are many different techniques to help reduce your stress and your body's reaction to stress. This list is just a few of the most common ones.

- Meditation
- Yoga/stretching
- Deep breathing exercises
- Exercise
- Gardening
- Reading
- Crafts/knitting/crochet
- Spending time with family

There are so many other options available. I watched a series on Disney+

titled "Limitless," and the very first episode talked about stress, what stress does to the body, and how you can start to minimize the effects of stress. The whole series follows Chris Hemsworth as he tries to find ways to increase longevity.

Sleep Hygiene

You may be wondering what sleep hygiene is.

It is creating and following a certain routine at night, designed to help you get ready for bed and go to sleep. This routine is completely up to you. You can determine how long you want to dedicate to it and what you want to include in it. But there are some guidelines that are highly recommended and some suggestions as well.

- *No screen time within an hour of going to bed.* This means putting your phone away and shutting your computer and TV off. This is important because the blue light that is emitted from the screens affects your body's ability to produce melatonin, your natural hormonal sleep aid. This is what helps you feel sleepy, fall asleep and stay asleep. If an hour is not doable, try for at least 30 minutes!
- *Do the same things in the same order every time.* This creates a pattern and a routine that your body will adapt to. When you start the routine, your body will then identify that it is time to get ready for bed. The more consistent you are with sticking with this routine, the easier it will be to fall asleep and stay asleep!

Quick Tip: keep your routine the same, regardless of if you have to work the next day or not. Go to bed at the same time and get up at the same time.

- *Limit caffeine after 5 pm.* If you are sensitive to the effects of caffeine, then you may want to limit it earlier in the day. Caffeine is a stimulant and is used to help provide energy. You don't want this interfering with your sleep because the quality of your sleep will suffer.

- *Limit liquid intake after 7 pm.* This simply reduces the number of trips you have to make to the bathroom in the middle of your sleep.
- *Keep your room cooler,* around 66 degrees. This may seem odd, but research has shown that you sleep better when the temperature of your room is cooler. I know when I have the temperature above 67, I don't sleep as well. I actually sleep best when it is around 65.
- *Invest in blackout curtains.* The darker the room, the better. It may seem obvious, but the more light there is, the less you are going to be able to sleep. You might be able to sleep, but your quality of sleep will be affected.

So how do you create a routine when you work nights? It isn't going to be like everyone else's. You will have one for the days that you are working and then one for when you are off. However you decide to create it, you need to make sure that you include it in your schedule. That ensures that you are giving yourself enough time to wind down before bed. My routine for going to bed after a shift is pretty simple and short. I have an hour's drive, which is some of my wind-down time. Once I get home, the only thing I do with my phone and watch is get them on the chargers and ensure that my alarm is on for the time I need it. I give my kids a hug and kiss (if they are home), brush my teeth, change into pajamas, and go to bed. On nights when I don't work, I give myself at least an hour to wind down. A big chunk of that time is spent snuggling with my twins (who are almost four at the time this is being written).

As with everything else, you have to figure out what works for you.

Family time

For some, family time is just as important, if not more important, than finding time to workout. If this is you, there is nothing wrong with that! Remember, exercise is not required in order to lose weight. Exercise is what will help to reshape your body. Yes, it can help to burn more fat, but you can lose weight without it. If family time is more important, simply make sure that when you are creating your schedule that you actually schedule in family time.

When my schedule gets really crazy (like when I schedule out time on my days off to work on my coaching business), I always make sure to have time reserved to spend with the family because being able to spend time with my family is important. I make sure that I have time throughout the week to have quality family time.

Quick tip: have a list of easy family activities you can do without having to go anywhere or even spend any money. Family games and movie nights are fun and relaxing ways to spend time together.

4

If I Can, So Can You!

I know that working night shift is hard, and it makes it harder to start a weight loss journey. But as you have seen in this book, it is completely possible. It just takes some creativity, commitment, and persistence. The weight isn't just going to melt off overnight. It didn't appear overnight, so it won't go away overnight. Have patience and keep going!

If you want to find out more about the specific nutrition programs I have used during my journey and the fitness programs that have helped to give me the results I have gotten, send me an email at prellfitness@gmail.com.

Thank you for taking the time to read this book. As a token of my appreciation, anyone who sends me an email will get my top 5 recipes that have helped me lose weight while enjoying amazing food!

Also by Melissa Prell

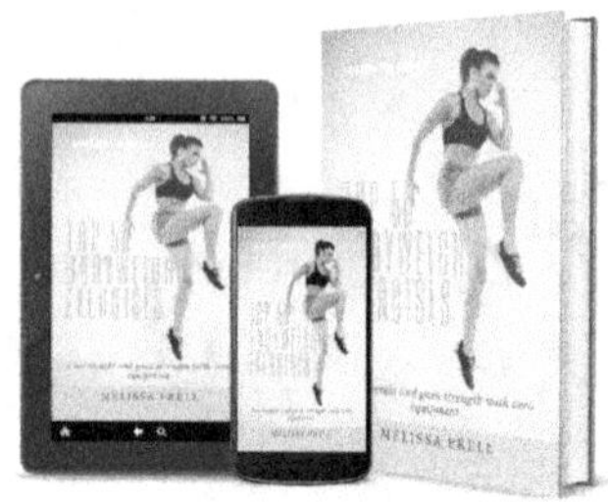

Top 50 Bodyweight Exercises: Low weight and gain strength with zero equipment

Learn how using just your bodyweight can help you lose weight and gain strength from the comfort of your home using no equipment. Three sample workouts provided at the end of the book for you to get started with! This would a great addition to help you battle the weightloss journey while working nightshift.